THE COLLAGEN DIET

Stimulate

metabolism

Anti-ageing from

within

Author: Melanie Krinz

copyright

Author: Melanie Krinz

Title: The Collagen Diet

© by Melanie Krinz, 2018

self publishing

<u>melanie.krinz@yahoo.de</u>

table of contents

FOREWORD

Collagen is responsible for firm skin and tightened facial contours. Various beauty products praise the anti-ageing effect of collagen and even celebrities swear by delicious shakes that build muscles, accelerate metabolism and keep the body firm.

How does collagen work? Where does the natural miracle cure come from and what functions does collagen have?

This guide deals with two questions: Why is collagen so important for our body and skin and how can you effectively integrate collagen uptake into your lifestyle so that you can benefit from all the positive properties of collagen.

Because if our body lacks collagen, the skin suffers from visible wrinkles and cellulite, hair and nails begin to break, joints and bones become noticeable of themselves. ☐

You will receive many effective tips

❖ for smooth, youthful and almost wrinkle-free skin
  ❖ for smooth bones and cartilage, so that your body can   draw from the full
                  every day
❖ how to improve your metabolism thanks to collagen
❖ how to build muscles thanks to collagen
❖ how to effectively declare war on cellulite
❖ how to regain a firm body shape
❖ valuable anti-ageing tips
❖ many recipes with collagen
❖ and much more...

You will live much healthier, more beautiful and recovered thanks to collagen. I promise.

WHAT IS COLLAGEN?

Collagen is not only the most important structural protein in the human body, but also the most abundant protein. Collagen is the raw material for our bones and skin.

Collagen fibres make up about one third of our protein content. The name collagen comes from Greek and means "glue-producing" and was formerly used as an adhesive in wood processing. Collagen also has a kind of adhesive function in the body, because the body uses it especially where tensile strength and resilience are important: collagen stabilizes our bones and cartilage as well as our teeth. Almost 60% of the connective tissue consists of the supporting protein, which can store up to 15 times its own mass of water. In the skin, collagen is essential for firmness and elasticity. Through targeted care, you can actively support a fresh and plump complexion.[1]

The collagen fibres consist of three individual long amino acid chains, which are twisted together spirally. It's called a triple helix.

Collagen contains the three amino acids glycine, proline and hydroxyproline, which the body itself needs to produce its own collagen. In general, these amino acids are otherwise difficult to absorb with food, unless you eat a lot of innards.

---

[1] https://www.vichy.at/le-vichy-mag/Kollagen-Anti-Aging-Power-gegen-Falten/vmag72904.aspx

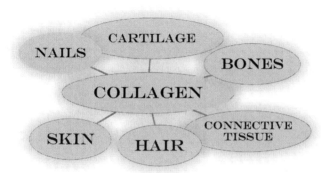

Collagen plays an important role in the entire body: in metabolism, in muscle building, in the formation of bones, hair, cartilage and above all skin. The connective tissue is supported by collagen fibres.

WHICH FACTORS ACCELERATE THE LOSS OF COLLAGEN?

Not only our age reduces the collagen in our body. Some factors play a role in how strongly collagen is degraded.

- ❖ Excessive exposure to sunlight,
- ❖ Smoking,
- ❖ Pollution,
- ❖ various pollutants,
- ❖ stress
- ❖ exaggerated sporting activities activate free radicals, which destroy the existing collagen.

❖ Hormone changes during menopause and aging reduce collagen formation.

In addition, various treatments that make the absorption of vitamins and minerals more difficult also influence collagen production.

WHAT IS THE EFFECT OF COLLAGEN?

Collagen supports the connective tissue of the body and gives it the structure and firmness seen and felt at a young age. Collagen keeps the skin young, smooth and above all firm.

The collagen fibres consist of rope-like structures which compress into fibres of high strength. They provide for elasticity and suppleness, which is indispensable for the elasticity of the skin.

Unfortunately, there is one factor everyone is exposed to: ageing. Collagen is broken down over time. Wrinkles and lines become visible, the tension of the skin inevitably gives way.

But the good news is: you can add the collagen by either taking collagen tablets, drinking collagen shakes or preparing collagen-rich food.

COLLAGEN ABSORPTION

Five years after menopause, women's falling estrogen levels mean that their skin contains up to 30 percent less collagen than at a young age. In order to prove the positive effects of collagen, many controlled clinical studies were conducted.[2]

Of particular importance are the studies by Zdzieblik et al. (2015), Cermak et al. (2012) and Hays et al. (2009), which dealt with the improvement of body balance, body composition and muscle mass.

As a result, they show positive results in muscle building and both decrease in fat mass, including in old age. Moskowitz (2000), Bruyère

---

[2] [Sibilla et al., 2015]

(2012), Flechsenhar and Sebastianelli (2007) as well as Oesser et al. (2016) could determine an improvement with joint pain, joint tension as well as on the cartilage tissue. In other studies, the administration of collagen led to positive effects on bone metabolism.[3]

Asserin et al. (2015), Inoue et al. (2016) and Proksch et al. (2015) have observed an improvement in skin hydration, a decrease in wrinkling, an improvement in skin texture and elasticity. Moreover, Schunck et al. (2015) showed a statistically significant improvement in cellulite in women of normal weight.[4]

There is no storage of collagen, because the

---

[3] [Moskowitz, 2000; Cúneo et al., 2010; Elam et al., 2015 and Kumar et al., 2015]
[4] https://allin-protein.com/pub/media/download/fachbeitra g/FACHBEITRAGKollagen.pdf

building blocks of collagen are immediately consumed by the body or built into the skin and joints. And in order for the body's own collagen to be produced at all, the body needs vitamin C.

There are capsules on the market for swallowing or protein powder for stirring into drinks or drinking ampoules. These consist of collagen peptides, which are tiny collagen particles that can be easily absorbed by the body.
If larger amounts of collagen or collagen hydrolysate are used, it is recommended to use them in drinking ampoules or powder form.
Collagen and collagen hydrolysate can be stirred into drinks or food.
Gelatine and collagen are obtained from animal raw materials such as cattle, pigs, chickens or fish. Those who do not eat pork products or are allergic to fish can switch to collagen from beef or chicken.

Collagen is neither vegetarian nor vegan. People who eat in this way can add other building blocks to joint and connective tissue problems, such as vegan amino acid mixtures and vegan glucosamine.[5]

What does that mean for us? Collagen uptake is very necessary after the age of 40 to prevent the body from slipping into the degradation process. The skin needs to look young and taut, the joints need collagen to remain supple and to continue to do their job.

---

[5]
https://www.vitamindoctor.com/naehrstoffe/sonstige-substanzen/kollagenkollagenhydrolysat/

COLLAGEN IS NOT EQUAL TO COLLAGEN

More than 20 variants of collagen are now known. The most important collagen types for us are collagen types I, II, III and IV.

Each type of collagen has its specific property in the human body.

There are different types of them. Collagen type II occurs in joints, type III in muscles, type I and III in skin. Simple gelatine is a mixture of type I, II and III collagen.

COLLAGEN TYPE I

Collagen type I is mainly found in skin and bones. But also tendons and ligaments consist of this collagen. This type of collagen occurs most frequently in the human body, we are talking about 90% of all collagen.

COLLAGEN TYPE II

While type I collagen is mainly found in bones and skin, type II collagen accounts for the majority of collagen found in cartilage. This is the most important difference between collagen type I and type II. The human cartilage consists of about 50% of this collagen type.

Collagen type II ensures a healthy, elastic joint cartilage composite. This collagen can also be found in the eyeball.

COLLAGEN TYPE III

Collagen III is an important component of reticular fibres, which in turn form the reticular connective tissue. This is mainly found in the lymphatic organs such as lymph nodes, spleen and tonsils.

Collagen type III in the tendons, connective tissue, bones and heart. It is particularly abundant in organs which, due to their function, must have a certain elasticity in everyday life. This naturally includes the skin, the lungs and the large arteries of our body.

The female uterus also contains a lot of type III collagen.

Collagen Type IV

Collagen type IV occurs mainly in the basement membrane. The basement membrane is a three-dimensional boundary layer in our body that surrounds muscle fibers, fat cells and nerve fibers.

Healthy joints

The supply of collagen seems to be very important for healthy joints and to reduce joint pain. The most common cause of unpleasant joint pain is a lack of collagen in the body. The body shows us what we need.

Collagen is particularly important for the strength of cartilage. It has therefore been investigated whether products containing collagen help with joint wear, arthrosis and promote cartilage formation.

In one study 108 volunteers with knee joint arthrosis were examined. They benefited from the intake of collagen. For 90 days they swallowed daily either:

- ❖ 20 milligrams of native collagen type II,
- ❖ a comparative medication (glucosamine, 375 milligrams, plus chondroitin sulfate, 300 milligrams)
- ❖ or a placebo.

The collagen was best for pain, joint stiffness and joint function, its effect was more than twice as high as that of glucosamine and chondroitin sulphate!

According to an evaluation of all available studies on this subject, collagen has a positive effect on pain. The data are less reliable if the joint function is restricted. Therefore, further studies will follow for confirmation.

In osteoarthritis, 10 to 40 milligrams of native collagen or 5,000 to 10,000 milligrams of collagen hydrolysate are used in studies.[6]

After a short time you will notice how much collagen will help your joints, cartilage and bones. Stay consistent and take your daily dose of collagen.

---

[6]
https://www.vitamindoctor.com/naehrstoffe/sonstige-substanzen/kollagenkollagenhydrolysat/

Stimulating the Metabolism with Collagen

Collagen can also positively stimulate the metabolism. Glycine plays a key role in this.

What is glycine?

Glycine is the smallest and simplest α amino acid and was first obtained in 1820 from gelatine, i.e. collagen hydrolysate. Glycine is not essential, can therefore be produced by the human organism itself and is an important component of almost all proteins and an important node in the metabolism.[7]

Glycine accounts for about one third of all amino acids found in collagen. Collagen in turn accounts for about 25% of all proteins in the body.

WHAT CAN GLYCINE DO?

- ❖ Glycine regulates the blood sugar level
- ❖ Glycine can reduce the increase in blood sugar levels by up to 50% in small amounts.

- ❖ Glycine improves sleep quality

  An evening intake of 3-5 g glycine before sleeping can improve the quality of sleep.

  ---

  [7]https://de.wikipedia.org/wiki/Glycin

Subjects who ate 3 g glycine before sleeping fell asleep faster and reached the first deep sleep phase earlier. In deep sleep, regeneration takes place mainly in the body. Then growth hormones are released, which support the repair of muscles and tissue damage in the body. Glycine may modulate NMDA receptors in the SCN (Suprachiasmatic Nucleus), which controls circadian rhythm.

- ❖ Glycine promotes the release of growth hormones

- ❖ Glycine promotes the release of STH (somatotropic hormone, growth hormone, HGH), which potentially positively affects basal endogenous STH production at night.

- ❖ Glycine improves memory performance

Glycine acts on the N-methyl D-aspartate receptor. This receptor plays a role in long-term potentiation (LTP). In LTP, information is transferred from short-term memory to long-term memory. The single oral administration of 100 mg glycine (in the form of bioglycine from Konopharma) facilitated the retrieval of previously learned information in the investigated group. In the older participants (> 50 years) the administration of glycine could also improve attention and concentration.

❖ Glycine reduces HbA1c, proinflammatory cytokines and increases interferon-γ in type 2 diabetics.

A daily intake of 5 g every 6 hours (20 g per day) for a variable duration of 3 - 56 months could reduce HbA1c in type 2 and type 1 diabetics and partly even normalize it.

❖ Glycine is given intravenously after liver transplantation to normalize the levels of transaminases and bilirubin. Glycine also influences the immune response and can help suppress rejection of the transplanted liver.

❖ Glycine inhibits inflammatory reactions

❖ Glycine inhibits the influx of calcium into leukocytes. As a result, PLA2 releases fewer fatty acids (e.g. arachidonic acid) and thus fewer prostaglandins are produced, which promote the inflammatory reaction. The reduced influx of calcium also leads to the formation of fewer cytokines such as TNFα and interleukins (IL-1, IL-6). Glycine can contribute to regulation and normalization in an overactive immune system. Glycine inhibits the activation of macrophages, the activation of nfκB and the formation of TNFα.

❖ Glycine inhibits proliferation of endothelial cells and smooth muscles

Due to its anti-inflammatory effect, glycine also counteracts the proliferation of endothelial cells and smooth muscle cells, which are increasingly formed during inflammatory reactions. Therefore, glycine can help with organ transplants and cardiovascular disease and support the regulation of uncontrolled angiogenesis (a characteristic of malignant tumors).

❖ Glycine improves blood circulation

Glycine improves the microcirculation and protects the cells against hypoxia. This effect is probably due to the inhibitory effect of glycine on nerve fibers that promote vasoconstriction and to the fact that vasoactive factors such as thromboxane A2, are less secreted.

❖ Glycine prevents cell destruction

Cells swell if they are damaged or have not been supplied with nutrients and oxygen for a long time. The swelling usually leads to the destruction of the cells. Glycine has a protective effect here. Glycine has been shown to protect renal tubule, liver and vascular cells from damage from hypoxia (oxygen deficiency), ischemia/reperfusion (no blood flow/reperfusion) and ATP deficiency. The mechanism is not exactly understood. Glycine is believed to stabilize the integrity of cell membranes and prevent the influx of ions that cause water and swelling.

❖ Glycine protects rats against toxic effects of methionine

The restriction of methionine in the diet can prolong the lifespan of rats. Methionine can promote the production of free radicals in the mitochondria of liver cells, thus damaging the mitochondrial membrane and leading to the destruction of liver cells.

❖ Glycine can normalize elevated blood pressure

Supplementation with glycine can help to normalize blood pressure by reducing inflammation and the positive effect on blood sugar regulation.

❖ Glycine (and L-arginine) help with reflux esophagitis (heartburn) in rats

❖ Glycine in combination with lactoferrin has an anti-inflammatory effect.

❖ Glycine protects against damage from shock caused by LPS (endotoxins)

- ❖ Glycine protects the gastric mucosa
- ❖ Glycine protects the gastric mucosa from irritation by aspirin and it improves the absorption of aspirin in the small intestine. Do not take aspirin together with individual amino acids!

- ❖ Glycine can reduce inflammation of the gums.[8]

- ❖ Glycine helps convert sugar into energy

Glycine is found mainly in foods that are rich in collagen. So tendons, connective tissue and bones. That's why bone broth is a good source of glycine. The long cooking process removes

---

[8] http://yourfunctionalmedicine.com/glycin-iss-nicht-nur-das-steak-teil-1/

collagen, other proteins, fats and minerals from the bone. These can thus be more easily absorbed in the digestive tract. The positive effects of glycine are another argument why it makes sense not only to eat muscle meat, but to use and appreciate the entire animal. If you don't get good quality bones and co. and still don't want to take a purely synthetic supplement, you can also cover your glycine needs by supplementing it with collagen hydrolysate. This should come best from animals which were kept as natural as possible (#grazing).

Other foods containing glycine are walnuts, pumpkin seeds or rice. Here, however, the proportion of glycine is much lower. 100 grams of walnuts contain 0.82 grams of glycine, 100 grams of gelatine contain about 23 grams of glycine. Glycine is also available in pure form, as powder. As its sweetening power is similar to sugar, it can also be used as a sugar substitute.[9]

Glycine, an important component of collagen, can have so many positive properties on our body and at the same time on our quality of life! Start integrating collagen into your lifestyle today, it pays off!

---

[9] http://yourfunctionalmedicine.com/glycin-iss-nicht-nur-das-steak-teil-1/

Increase muscle growth with collagen

Collagen peptides, which naturally have a lower content of branched chain amino acids, have so far only been studied to a limited extent. Nevertheless, one study showed that both muscle mass and strength could be increased by the administration of bioactive collagen peptides in combination with strength training compared to placebo [Zdzieblik et al 2015].

One explanation for the effectiveness of these collagen peptides could be that collagen peptides have a better nitrogen balance than whey protein [Hays et al 2009]. In addition, collagen peptides are rich in glycine and arginine, from which creatine phosphate, an important source of energy for muscle work, is formed in the body [Berdanier 2015].

Glycine also has many important physiological effects and, although it is not an essential amino acid, can become essential under certain circumstances [Razak et al 2017].

For example, people with obesity or diabetes have a disturbed glycine metabolism [Adeva-Andany et al 2018].

Glycine is extremely important in stabilizing the collagen superhelix and a deficiency may manifest itself in the functionality of blood vessels and other collagen structures such as connective tissue [Adeva-Andany 2018, Razak et al 2017].

The close interaction of muscle tissue with surrounding connective tissue makes a connection plausible. The use of bioactive collagen peptides reduces pain in joints caused by intensive training [Zdzieblik et al 2017].

In a double-blind, randomized study, Zdzieblik et al investigated the influence of bioactive collagen peptides in combination with strength training on fat-free muscle mass and muscle strength in older volunteers with age-related muscle atrophy (sarcopenia) over three months [Zdzieblik et al 2015].

Included were healthy men over 65 years of age with sarcopenia, normal western diet and adequate protein intake.

53 volunteers underwent intensive strength training three times a week for 60 minutes over a period of 12 weeks.

- ❖ 26 received daily 15 g bioactive collagen peptides as powder dissolved in 250 ml water,
- ❖ 27 people 15 g placebo (silicon dioxide).

On training days the powder should be taken within one hour after training, on training days at the same time if possible.

After three months, an increase in fat-free muscle mass, muscle strength and bone mass as well as a decrease in fat mass could be achieved in all groups with an almost unchanged body weight, which suggests a pronounced training effect.

In the verum group, however, these effects were significantly more pronounced than in the placebo group, which suggests a positive effect of the bioactive collagen peptides.[10]

---

[10] https://bioaktive-kollagenpeptide.de/wirkungen-muskulatur/

This means that collagen has a great influence on muscle growth. That is why it makes sense to absorb collagen in everyday life.

Reduce cellulite and stretch marks with collagen

If the skin loses its elasticity, it automatically contains less collagen. It becomes thinner and cellulite and stretch marks are more clearly visible.

There are 3 reasons for cellulite:

❖ Soft skin and connective tissue
❖ Too much fat
❖ connective tissue fibres

Soft skin and connective tissue is unfortunately the worst to treat. Often creams and other remedies are used against it. However, once the skin has reached a certain "softness" stage, it can no longer be treated effectively. In the aging process, tissue becomes softer as collagen is lost and elastic fibres are broken down.

But cellulite is not just a question of weight!

Under the skin there are connective tissue fibres, which can contract in the course of life. It is best to imagine a string that pulls the skin downwards in some places - this causes the unattractive dents on the skin surface.[11]

---

[11] https://www.theaesthetics.at/3-ursachen-von-cellulite/

If the body can build up more collagen through dietary supplementation, it becomes more even, smoother and more elastic again. This is where collagen effectively helps to get the cellulite problem under control from the inside out.

Tip: Forget all expensive anti-cellulite products! Invest in gelatine powder or collagen drinks to drink, because that really helps.

COLLAGEN UPTAKE IN FOOD

In addition to the protein sources mentioned above, which have a high calcium content and thus push the energy metabolism, it is more than advantageous to integrate gelatine or collagen hydrolysate into the diet. After 2 to 3 months you will experience the difference visibly and perceptibly on your own body!

Collagen peptides have an almost neutral taste and smell. Due to their low molecular weight, collagen peptides are easily digestible and can be easily absorbed and distributed in the human body.

COLLAGEN HYDROLYSATE

A hydrolysate is the product of hydrolysis. Protein or protein hydrolysates are often used in sports and sports medicine. The "free" amino acids contained in it are more easily absorbed by the body than the proteins themselves, so the nutrient supply of muscle tissue is accelerated.[12]

Production of collagen hydrolysate: When collagen is heated with acids and alkalis, smaller fragments, so-called collagen peptides, are formed. In contrast to gelatine, gelatine hydrolysates in water do not form a gel but are liquid. Collagen hydrolysate: Collagen and its hydrolysate are low in calories and even replace

---

[12] https://de.wikipedia.org/wiki/Hydrolysat

part of the fat and salt in light products. Collagen is broken down in the intestine and the building blocks and smaller fragments are absorbed. Collagen hydrolysate is already "pre-digested"; the fragments are available to the body after only four hours.

Producing collagen hydrolysate is even more complex than producing gelatine. In addition, the collagen peptides are treated with enzymes until the desired end product is obtained.

Collagen & Gelatine

Gelatine consists of 90% collagen and is very low in calories.

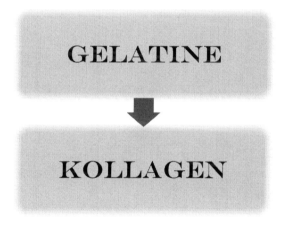

The known gelatine is nothing more than an effective collagen solution. It is inexpensive and can be found in almost every shop. Simple gelatine is a mixture of collagen type I, II and III.

In most cases, almost only muscle meat is eaten. The bones or cartilage are not used in the fast-moving kitchen. The other "part" of the animal, which is found in bones and cartilage, is simply missing: gelatine. It consists of glycine, proline and hydroxyproline. All three amino acids are lacking in the end consumer due to the one-sided consumption of meat in everyday life.

Gelatine is therefore an important building block for rebalancing this imbalance. Not only to ensure a firm and young connective tissue, but also to guarantee a complete amino acid uptake. The body just likes balance.

In this context, collagen hydrolysate is equivalent to gelatine. It is extracted from collagen. The structural protein collagen also provides a firm and flexible connective tissue.

In contrast to gelatine, hydrolysate does not have any gelling properties. In collagen hydrolysate we find short amino acid chains, so-called peptides, which are biologically highly available. Peptides can be absorbed into the bloodstream through the intestinal wall.[13]

---

[13] https://www.fit-and-fresh.com/effektiv-den-stoffwechsel-ankurbeln-1x1/

Collagen in skin creams

Creams and serums reach the surface of the skin, especially the horny layer, and are mainly effective here.

However, as a rule they do not reach the deep layers of the skin, i.e. where the causes of the aging processes can be found. Only cosmetic acids such as fruit acid, glycolic acid or mandelic acid can do this. These work deeper than any skin cream.

COLLAGEN & HYALURONIC ACID

Collagen and hyaluronic acid are naturally present in the body and form a close partnership in the deeper skin layer, the dermis.

"The skin forms both. The basis is the collagen framework, which gives the skin its elasticity. It must be intact in order for the hyaluronic acid to spread well in the skin," explains Dr. Jan-Christoph Kattenstroth, Medical Director of the pharmaceutical manufacturer Quiris Healthcare. However, UV light and, with increasing age, the decrease in certain hormones affect the symbiosis.

How can we ensure that collagen and hyaluron production continues? With anti-aging creams and serums that contain these active ingredients? *"No. The idea that collagen or high-molecular hyaluronic acid from creams penetrates into the dermis and thus stimulates collagen metabolism has not been proven in scientific studies,"* says Prof. Dr. Martina Kerscher, dermatologist and cosmetics scientist at the University of Hamburg. What they can do, however, is to moisturize and pampers the epidermis, the uppermost layer of the skin, making the complexion softer, finer and more supple for several hours.

They also strengthen the skin's barrier and make it more resistant to environmental influences. With collagen, the skin feels better and looks more beautiful as it shrinks slightly as the product dries, eliminating small bumps and dents. Hyaluron in turn binds moisture in the skin and improves elasticity.

"If collagen production is promoted, more hyaluronic acid is generated. A win-win situation, so to speak," says Dr. Kattenstroth.

But how does it work?

"It is comparable to a key-lock principle," said Prof. Kerscher, who carried out a study with the collagen drink Elasten. "The *collagen peptides are absorbed through the intestine, where they are split into di- and tripeptides, which are distributed through the blood circulation in the body. They also reach the dermis and stimulate the connective tissue metabolism of the skin, i.e. more collagen and hyaluron is produced.*"

THE EFFECT: After absorption into the tissue, the highest concentration was detected in the skin. After twelve weeks, elasticity, firmness, firmness and resilience were improved. Whether you prefer creams, fillers or drinks is a matter of taste. What is certain is that every treatment should be garnished with UV protection. Prevention is the best aftercare.[14]

---

[14] https://www.harpersbazaar.de/beauty/haut-hyaluron-kollagen

COLLAGEN PROMOTES HEALTHY SLEEP

The sleep-promoting qualities of collagen come from the high glycine content of the protein. Research showed that people with sleep disorders fell asleep faster, went into deep sleep faster and reported less daytime sleepiness the next day. You were also able to concentrate better. This is another indication that they were more rested.

In another study, participants who took collagen before going to sleep were less tired and had a clearer head the next day. A third study found that collagen does not contribute to daytime fatigue, even if you use it during the day.

The glycine contained in collagen promotes healthy sleep. Collagen consists of about 33 percent glycine, one of the most abundant amino acids in collagen. Glycine is a non-essential amino acid, so it can be formed in the human body itself. Glycine is important for healthy skin generation, the formation of hair all over the body and the development of cartilage, especially joint cartilage.

Take it an hour before going to bed. You can combine it very well with melatonin. Melatonin is a hormone produced in the pineal gland, a tiny part of the diencephalon. This gland controls the day-night rhythm of the body via the release of melatonin. If light falls into the eye during the day, the release of the hormone into the blood is stopped. At night, in the absence of light, melatonin is released from the stores and can unfold its sleep-promoting effect.

Older people suffering from insomnia have lower nocturnal melatonin levels than their peers with undisturbed sleep. Advertising attributes fantastic effects to the body's own messenger substance: The pineal gland hormone is classified in the group of radical scavengers; similar effects to vitamin E are said to occur.

It is therefore intended to combat the development of diseases as diverse as cancer and atherosclerosis. An inhibitory influence on the sex hormone balance is also suspected.

The body produces less melatonin with increasing age. This circumstance led to the assumption that melatonin influences aging itself as well as age-related diseases.

In rats and mice, reduced melatonin secretion is directly associated with an accelerated aging process. By preventing cell damage by neutralizing free radicals and at the same time strengthening the immune response, melatonin may reduce signs of aging.

However, the age-related reduction of nocturnal melatonin secretion could also be a consequence of the aging process and not its cause. So far, no studies have shown that melatonin affects the aging process in humans. However, several studies showed clear indications of a sleep-promoting effect. It is therefore possible that the substance has sufficient potential to be used in sleep disorders. However, studies showing which patients could benefit from which dosage are still lacking. There are very contradictory data on the relationship between melatonin and tumor development. Most studies indicate a protective effect of melatonin.

Low levels of melatonin were found in women with breast cancer and men with prostate cancer. Also, the half-life of melatonin is too short to allow therapeutic application. Research projects are currently underway to find a further development of melatonin with regard to a longer half-life.[15]

---

[15]
https://www.netdoktor.at/therapie/melatonin
-8763

COMBINATION COLLAGEN & VITAMIN C

Vitamin C is not only a basic requirement for collagen synthesis, but also a stimulant. This shows a current study at human Hautfibroblasten in which it could be proven that the long-term treatment with vitamin C over 5 days the synthesis of collagen I and IV improved clearly.

Vitamin C not only promotes a healthy and firm connective tissue through collagen synthesis, but is also involved in the formation of elastin, fibronectin and proteoglycan.

Vitamin C also has Einfluss on the concentration of hyaluronic acid, which binds a lot of water and gives the skin a youthful appearance. Vitamin C helps protect hyaluronic acid from the rapid enzymatic degradation triggered by inflammatory mediators and an acidic environment.

Unfortunately, vitamin C blood levels decrease with age. This has serious consequences for aging, as damage from reactive oxygen compounds (ROS) plays an important role in aging processes, and vitamin C is one of the most effective natural antioxidants.

A study of 95 men and 122 women aged 12 to 96 observed a clear age-related decrease in vitamin C blood levels. From the age of 40, the average vitamin C blood value decreases in women.

In addition to its essential function in collagen synthesis, vitamin C is important for immune and nerve function. These cells have the highest vitamin C concentrations in humans.

An undersupply is accompanied by an increased susceptibility to infections and depressive mood. The latter is explained by the involvement of vitamin C in the synthesis of important neurotransmitters (norepinephrine, adrenaline, dopamine and serotonin). Other early symptoms of vitamin C deficiency are fatigue and weakness.[16]

---

[16] https://www.kosmetischemedizin-online.de/vitamin-c-ein-wichtiger-baustein-der-bildung-straffer-kollagenfasern/

Regeneration at night thanks to collagen

Collagen, taken in the evening, supports the regeneration of the body.

A shake with collagen in the evening, which contains about 3 grams of glycine, promotes sleep quality and increases the regeneration of the body. This has a positive effect on mental and spiritual performance the very next day.

Foods that promote the formation of collagen

Let's start with the meats. Meat is an excellent supplier of collagen. In particular, the following varieties are recommended:

- ➢ **cow meat**
- ➢ **fryers**
- ➢ **goat meat**
- ➢ **beef**
- ➢ **venison**

Pork meat, especially the legs of the pork meat, also called "**knuckles**", contain a lot of useful collagen. **Tripe, bone** and other parts of the pig also contain a lot of protein and collagen.

Although fish contains less collagen than meat, it also provides other important proteins, especially those found in scales.

Fatty fish such as **salmon & tuna** also contain Omega 3, which protects the fat membrane around the skin cells. This allows you to make your skin firmer and more elastic.

Red fruit & vegetables, such as apples, **strawberries, cherries, beetroot, tomatoes, red peppers, all berries** contain lycopene / lycopene. This is a substance that has an antioxidant effect and promotes the formation of collagen.

Vitamin C is essential for the production of collagen. This can be found especially in the following fruits: **Orange, lemon, kiwi, grapefruit, mango, pineapple**...

Vegetables also help in the production of collagen. **Cabbage, cucumbers, aubergines, kale, endive salad** or **spinach ensure** a successful supply of collagen.

Celery, green and black olives, garlic & onion and tofu contain valuable sulphur compounds which also promote the production of collagen.

The Collagen Killer

Smoking is the collagen killer No. 1. Apart from alcohol and excessive sunbathing, smoking is very harmful for the human cell and also for healthy collagen production. This can be seen in large bags under the eyes, flaccid cheeks and wrinkles around the mouth and nose. These characteristics are very pronounced in smokers. The skin colour of smokers is also usually rather pale.

Nicotine is responsible for narrowing the blood vessels and thus restricting healthy blood circulation. One cigarette is enough to greatly reduce the blood flow in the skin for more than an hour! The nicotine makes the skin age faster, as collagen and elastic fibres of the skin are disturbed in their function.

The proteins that normally ensure a healthy skin structure are destroyed by smoking.

Several processes are responsible for the increased formation of wrinkles in the smoker's skin. Tobacco smoke inhibits the formation of new collagen fibres in the dermis and at the same time promotes the breakdown of collagen and elastin fibres. Thus the finely tuned system of building up and dismantling the fibres gets out of balance. In addition, the epidermis of smokers contains less water than that of non-smokers, which in turn contributes to the increased formation of wrinkles.

The longer you smoke, the faster the skin ages. The skin of smokers who consume 20 cigarettes a day is already ten years older in middle age than that of non-smokers!

The toxic substances from tobacco smoke also damage the mucous membranes of the mouth. Smoking is a significant risk factor for changes in the oral cavity and inflammation of gums and gums.[17]

The enzyme MMPs (Matrix Metalloproteinases) accelerates the aging of the skin. Scientific studies show that body cells exposed to tobacco smoke produce significantly larger amounts of this enzyme. Nicotine unfortunately also influences the breakdown of the tissue that produces new collagen for the regenerating skin and in this way ensures its resilience and elasticity.

---

[17] https://www.haut.de/gesichtshaut-altert-durch-rauchen/

Laboratory tests have shown that collagen production decreases by up to 40 percent. By slowing down the natural skin renewal processes, the dead, horny skin flakes remain on the skin surface for longer. A thicker horny layer is formed, which makes the skin look grey and tired.[18]

The renunciation of smoking is without doubt an important contribution to skin health. If you are considering stopping nicotine use, you must be patient. Skin support tissue damaged by the unhealthy blue haze takes time to renew. Of course, this does not happen overnight, but you will notice a visible difference after only a few weeks.

---

[18] http://www.beauty.at/skin/facts/Trend-Reports-Die-Haut-raucht-mit.html

RECIPES

WITH

COLLAGEN

RECIPES WITH COLLAGEN

You can fill your food very easily with collagen. It's not difficult, and the result will be impressive: Your joints will become much smoother, the connective tissue much firmer. This will also visibly change your skin structure, so that wrinkles will significantly decrease. However, you should build the collagen supply into your food intake stably and really over maintain.

Gelatine is certainly the main carrier of collagen. Gelatine is a mixture of substances that mainly contains collagen, but also other substances and can bind water well. Gelatine is produced, for example, when bones are boiled and the collagen contained in them is released. Gelatine ensures a healthy digestive system by regulating the production of gastric acid and renewing the mucous membrane of the stomach.[19]

I have compiled recipes for you that are easy to install and can be used daily without having to change much of your favourite food.

A lot of collagen contains pieces of meat with a lot of connective tissue. These are knuckles, shoulder pieces.

CONNECTIVE TISSUE - MUSCLE FLESH

In cattle meat (as in any other animal), a basic distinction is made between two types of meat: short fibrous muscle pieces and pieces with long fibrous muscles and a lot of connective tissue.

---

[19] https://www.paleo360.de/gesunde-ernaehrung/iss-mehr-gelatine-superfood-collagen/

Short-fibre muscles develop in cattle in all those places where the cow hardly needs muscle strength. This is above all the back, which remains permanently in the same position. The pieces lying there consist of very short-fibred muscles, which are naturally tender - they could also be eaten raw, so soft and friable is their structure, because they hardly have to do any work.

The muscles of the limbs required by cattle for locomotion consist of long fibres and stable connective tissue with a high proportion of collagen. These are building blocks that can withstand high resistances, and these muscle parts are correspondingly tough in their raw form.

Fry filet, roast beef, entrecote or hip in the pan, denature the protein strands that come into contact with heat immediately. They contract and thus push the water contained in the muscle outwards. Strongly denatured muscle meat is grey, dry and culinary no longer usable.

In short roasting, the aim is therefore to expose as few areas of the meat as possible to excessive heat in order to prevent large parts from completely denaturing and drying out.

That is also the reason why medium or rare cooked meat still tastes juicy and a well-done fried steak does not. This is about minutes or even seconds, a few degrees more or less.

Short fibrous muscle parts are tender and juicy, but only as long as they are not heated too high. Those parts, that support the movement apparatus of the animal, are of completely different condition and behave therefore also differently with the roast. The connective tissue with its high collagen content is central.

Tendons and cartilage are also made of collagen. This collagen slowly transforms into gelatine during cooking - this soft, slimy mass that is also known from cake glazes. This gelatine in turn is responsible for the fact that a piece of braised meat does not dry out, but becomes juicier and juicier as the cooking time continues.

The transformation of hard collagen into creamy gelatine takes time and a higher temperature than with short frying. While a fillet dries out completely from 60 degrees, the collagen conversion process only starts at 65 degrees and takes several hours at this temperature. At higher temperatures between 70 and 80 degrees, the process is a little faster, but at the same time other denaturation processes in the meat start, which prevent a perfect result with braised meat.

In practice, this means either cooking "sous-vide" at +65 degrees or meticulously making sure that the stewing liquid does not begin to simmer when stewing in a pot. Parts like bow, club, mayor's piece etc. do not only consist of collagen - they also contain muscle tissue, which behaves in the same way on contact with heat as the muscle parts of the short roast piece. The muscle strands contract and push the water out of the cells.

But unlike filet & co., this meat juice is not lost: gelatine has the ingenious property that it can bind ten times its own weight in liquid. It absorbs the water squeezed out by the muscles and preserves the juiciness of the braised meat.

Since the collagen conversion process takes hours, parts with a high connective tissue content also benefit from a long cooking time. So if a restaurant advertises "6 hours of braised ox cheeks", then there is a good reason. And to be honest, eight would be even better. The fact that such braised pieces can contain an extremely high amount of gelatine can also be seen from the brew that is produced during braising. When you let it cool, the sauce freezes like jell-o. No wonder: The main ingredient of jelly is... right - gelatine!

If one declares meatcuts as a "piece of braised meat", one has to look at them twice in the meantime. "Modern cutting techniques ensure that even pieces rich in collagen and sinewy parts can still be made into short roasts," says meat expert Christoph Grabowski. Best example: The flat shoulder.

Long used only as a sauerbraten cut, butchers today cut two steaks by removing the middle tendon. In the eyes of connoisseurs, the so-called "Flat Iron", which is then created, even competes with the fillet and is perfectly suited for short frying due to its texture and without the internal tendon.[20]

---

[20]

https://www.fleischglueck.de/magazin/kollagen-gelatine-schmoren/

Bone broth with collagen

Bone broth is considered a true superfood, because collagen is released from the bones when it boils, it has healing properties. It calms aching bones and muscles, fights infection successfully and improves your skin, as there is a lot of collagen in the broth. The energy level is also naturally increased.

In addition to the unique taste of a bone broth and its versatile use in the kitchen, bone broth is an excellent source of certain amino acids and minerals. It offers a lot of health benefits. **No bag of soup can be compared to a homemade bone broth!**

When making your own bone broth, be sure to buy only the best chicken or beef from sustainable agriculture. It's definitely worth it!

Bovine collagen is a naturally occurring protein found in the cartilage, bones and skin of cows, and is similar to what is in your own body. There is also something known as Type I and III collagen, which are the main components in your skin, nails, hair, tendons, ligaments, muscles and bones, as well as your teeth, gums, eyes and blood vessels.

Bovine collagen provides the aforementioned glycine, an immune nourishing amino acid necessary to build DNA and RNA strands, and one of the three amino acids that make up creatine, which promotes the growth of healthy muscles and helps produce energy during exercise, as well as "proline", another amino acid critical to the body's own collagen production.[21]

You can buy bones of beef or chicken in the supermarket or at the butcher's, just ask your butcher. Instead of always eating only the fillet of beef, you can take a holistic approach here. It's good for the wallet, too.[22]

Bone stock is very easy to boil down. So you can cook on stock and you always have a homemade conche broth at hand. For bone broth, boil for 120 minutes at 100 degrees.

---

[21]
https://german.mercola.com/sites/articles/arc hive/2017/10/10/kollagen-besser-haut.aspx
[22]
https://www.paleo360.de/rezepte/knochenbru ehe/

Ingredients

500 g bones of beef - especially marrow bones

1.5 to 2.0 litres of water

Soup vegetables

Garlic

Salt and pepper to taste

Lovage, laurel leaf as desired

Peel the carrot and onions and cut into coarse pieces. Wash soup vegetables, e.g. celeriac, leek, parsley and cut into coarse pieces. Crush and peel the garlic. Put the bone in a large pot and roast without fat. Add the pre-cut vegetables to the bones and continue roasting together. Fill bones and vegetables with water until everything is covered. Let simmer for 3-4 hours. After about 3 hours, remove the marrow from the bones and continue cooking. Pour the bone stock through a sieve into another pot. Season to taste.

Tip: the higher the proportion of bones, tendons and skin in the bone broth, the more gelatine can dissolve and the more intense the typical meat taste in the broth. A good broth gelatinized at refrigerator temperatures.

ASPIC WITH CHICKEN

Aspic is another name for jelly made from meat or fish. The word 'aspic' was borrowed in the 19th century from the French 'aspic', 'jelly, meat sauce, stock', the origin of which is uncertain.

To prepare aspic dishes, small portion moulds made of metal or glass are strongly cooled, poured with spiced jelly which is still just liquid, cooled again until a thin coat has solidified on the vessel wall, the remaining jelly poured off, small slices of truffles, carrots, cucumbers or similar decoratively inlaid, the ice-cold filling made of meat, fish, seafood, hard-boiled eggs or even vegetables put in and everything covered with liquid jelly with liquid jelly. After the jelly has solidified completely in the refrigerator, the moulds are briefly dipped into hot water and the aspike is put on plates.[23]

INGREDIENTS:

WATER

CHICKEN PIECES FROM THE THIGH

SOUP VEGETABLES

GELATINE

The chicken legs are placed in cold water, brought to the boil and the rising protein is strained with a ladle. When all the free floating protein has been removed, pickle the vegetables, reduce heat and cook for about 2 hours.

---

[23] https://de.wikipedia.org/wiki/Aspik

Strain the vegetable stock, let it get very hot again, dissolve the corresponding amount of gelatine in it. No more cooking! Season to taste. The brew should now be slightly salted and seasoned to taste, then after cooling it is perfect in taste.

Peel the meat from the bone, cut it and spread it with the boiled carrots in small bowls. Carefully empty the vegetable stock with the gelatine. Allow to cool.

Braised Pieces of Meat

Ingredients:

Pieces of meat with a lot of

connective tissue, natural

gelatine - knuckles of pork,

oxtail

Soup vegetables

Tomato puree

Broth

First season large pieces of meat well with salt and pepper, then sauté vigorously. When the meat is fried, take it out of the roaster, add vegetables such as onions, carrots and celery to the hot fat and roast it well. A good portion of tomato paste can also be roasted. Then add the meat again and deglaze with wine or broth.

Fish in aspic

Ingredients:

1 whole fish or 2 fillet pieces

(salmon, lake trout, trout, pike,

zander)

Root vegetables

Bay leaf, peppercorns, salt

Gelatine

Preparation

Prepare a vegetable stock from the roots and the spices. Cut the fish fillets into pieces about 3 cm wide and place them carefully in the broth. You can also add the fillets as a whole, but you should cut them into smaller pieces after cooking. - After about 15 minutes the fish is cooked. Remove the fish pieces carefully and put them into a glass mould. Decorate with cut carrots and peas.

Strain the vegetable stock, let it get very hot again, dissolve the corresponding amount of gelatine in it. No more cooking! Season to taste. The brew should now be slightly salted and seasoned to taste, then after cooling it is perfect in taste. Pour the gelatine stock carefully over the fish pieces and allow to set.

COLLAGEN CUBES

Collagen cubes can be made at home. You need animal pieces rich in collagen, such as chicken feet. The chicken feet are particularly rich in natural collagen, and the brew becomes really "sticky". You can get them from any butcher.

The finished collagen cubes are easy to freeze. They are **odourless** and **tasteless**, so they can be used in any sauce or soup. Pour the finished brew into ice cube bags. This is a good way to portion the collagen-containing brew.

INGREDIENTS:

Cold water

Chicken feet and/or knuckle of

pork

Pour cold water over the meat or animal pieces
and cook for a very long, really long time until a
gel-like liquid is formed and the meat fibres fall
off the conches. Add water again and again.
Strain the finished broth, allow to cool slightly
and then carefully fill into ice cube bags.

Japanese soup "hub mono"

The Japanese are real experts on collagen in food.

"Hub" means stew. A traditional "hub" consists of abundant ingredients of vegetables, fish and meat that are cooked together in a broth, and these dishes are known for their great nutritional value. For this purpose, the broth is enriched with collagen.

The collagen stew boom in Japan began when a restaurant introduced a "beauty hub" containing collagen derived from chicken bones. The collagen soup was sold as the elixir of youth. Other restaurants picked up on this trend and collagen-based stews could be found all over the country within a very short time.

INGREDIENTS:

1 L WATER OR DASHI

8 SHIITAKE DRIED

75 G MISO

1/2 KABOCHA

1/2 DAIKON SMALL

3 SMALL TARO

2 SPRING ONIONS

1 CARROT

1/4 CHINESE CABBAGE

1/2 PCK SHIMEJI

2 UDON PORTIONS

SHICHIMI TŌGARASHI

Shiitake overnight or for at least five hours in water. This makes the broth. Alternatively, only Dashi can be used. Dissolve Miso in the broth.

Squeeze out the shiitake, halve and remove the strand. Peel the pumpkin (the shell of the Kabocha is also edible) and cut into bite-sized pieces.

Halve Daikon and carrot lengthwise and cut into pieces. Quarter the taro lengthwise and if necessary also cut it into pieces. Cut the spring onions into 3-4cm long pieces. Cut Chinese cabbage and remove strand of Shimeji.

Put the mushrooms and vegetables with the broth in the pot. Let simmer for about 10 minutes.

Add the Udon noodles and simmer again for about 10 minutes.

Serve hot and sprinkle with Shichimi tōgarashi to taste.[24]

---

[24] http://bento-daisuki.de/rezept/hoto-nabe/

Vegan Collagen Protein Shake

Ingredients for 1 collagen drink:

250 ml coconut water or still

mineral water

2 tbsp vegan protein powder

1 handful Kiwi

1 handful strawberries

1 banana

2 sheets gelatine, dissolved

Preparation

Blend all ingredients in a mixer for about 30 seconds until the collagen drink is velvety and creamy.

FRUITY JELL-O

INGREDIENTS:

500 ML FRUIT JUICE

6 SHEETS GELATINE

Place the gelatine in cold water for about 10 minutes. Each leaf of gelatine needs its own deep plate with cold water, otherwise clumps can form.

Then do not squeeze the gelatine too much and place it in a pot. Heat the gelatine slightly in the pot and let it melt while stirring constantly. Attention: The gelatine must not boil, otherwise it will not become solid after cooling down. Now slowly add the juice while stirring constantly. Mix well until the gelatine is completely mixed with the juice. refrigeration points and after a few hours enjoy.

TIP: If you need to go fast, use gelatine jelly babies.

Low Fat Dessert with Fruit

Ingredients

250 g strawberries

250 g curd cheese

200 ml cream

50 g sugar

1 pck. cream stiffener

5 sheets gelatine

1 sachet vanilla sugar

1 LEMON(S) - PEEL, GRATED

Strawberries puree. Mix the quark, sugar and grated lemon zest. Add the strawberries.

Dissolve the gelatine and add to the quark mixture. Whip cream with cream stiffener + vanilla sugar until stiff and mix with quark. Keep cool.

Gelatine - Face Mask

Ingredients:

2-3 leaves gelatine

5ml hot water

10 drops lemon juice

Dissolve gelatine in hot water, add fresh lemon juice, wait about 10 minutes and apply face mask to cleansed skin with a brush. When the mask becomes firm, rinse with warm water. Use 2 times a week.

Further Anti-Ageing Tips

Against Wrinkles

Dinner Canceling

If the cells slag from the inside, the best care did
not help. The current state of knowledge is that
intermittent fasting not only breaks down toxic
metabolic residues, but also stimulates the
regeneration of healthy cells. Here it helps to
take a daily break from eating for 14 hours, for
example overnight. During this time, important
regeneration processes take place that stimulate
healthy cell renewal.

It also stimulates the breakdown of fat. Nutritionists recommend not having dinner once or twice a week. The results are not only noticeable on the scale.

You can combine the Dinner Canceling with the collagen diet very well. Paint dinner, take collagen tablets or a collagen shake instead. The collagen unfolds its effectiveness overnight to the Dinner Canceling. You'll be surprised at how that makes itself felt.

Avoid sugar

In the anti-ageing fight, high-quality cosmetic brands rely on active ingredients that can prevent the "glycolisation" of the skin. The adhesion of the cells by excessive amounts of sugar is inhibited in such a way that ultimately the formation of wrinkles is promoted.

So it is much smarter not to let the unhealthy sugar into the organism in the first place. The less sugar in the blood and thus in the skin layers circulates, the longer the body remains beautiful and wrinkle-free, from head to toe!

MASSAGES: THE PAMPERING PROGRAM FOR CELL REGENERATION

The better your connective tissue and skin layers are supplied with blood, the tighter they will appear. That is why regular plucking massages belong to the proven anti-ageing tips. They tighten the stomach, as well as legs, bottom and upper arms. Massages ensure that the skin is well supplied with blood right down to the deep layers. Ideal is a massage daily after showering. Oils or creams that increase blood circulation can help to further increase success.

TIGHT CONTOURS THANKS TO REGULAR MOVEMENT

The silhouette of the body must be defined with gymnastics. That doesn't change much. This is exhausting and unfortunately indispensable. Therefore my tip to you: Get into a sport that you enjoy and that also spreads a good mood. It's no use practicing a sport that only creates frustration. Sooner or later you won't do it. Tightening exercises include spinning, aerobics,

Tae Bo or stretching. The sporting activity stimulates the cell activity and acts like a fountain of youth on the whole body.

My tip to you: When you finish your sports unit in the evening, you can spread your evening meal afterwards.

EXFOLIATION

In my book "Wrinkle-free thanks to fruit acid" I describe exactly how cosmetic acids such as fruit acid, mandelic acid or glycolic acid work. You're not just peeling your skin. Their effect on collagen production is impressive. Cosmetic fruit acids can stimulate the cell activity and thus the skin cells produce more collagen. No skin cream can do that, not even the most expensive in the world.

Pay attention to facial expressions

Facial movements that you make frequently cause wrinkles more quickly when your skin loses elasticity. If you often pinch your eyes together or pull your brows together, the frown lines and small wrinkles around your eyes are more likely to appear in early years.

The same applies if you drink drinks with straws. There are wrinkles threatening over the lip, which really make every woman look much older.

But you should never stifle laughter, please. Happy and with a few more wrinkles it lives much better than unhappy and with fewer wrinkles.

SLEEP YOUNG

Sleep is one of the most effective and natural anti-ageing measures. While we slumber deeply and firmly, there is a lot going on in our body. During sleep, the body produces large amounts of the very important growth hormone HGH, which is responsible for the division and renewal of cell tissue.

In addition to a sufficient amount of sleep, about seven hours should be enough, the physical condition during sleep is also crucial. The HGH release can only take place if it is not slowed down by an increased insulin level! Only those who keep their insulin levels throttled about three hours before sleep sleep sleep sleep young. That means: about three hours before you go to bed, you should avoid food and especially sweetened drinks.

ANTI-AGEING FACIAL EXERCISES

The muscle tissue lies close under the skin. The firmer it is, the firmer the skin will look. This applies not only to the body, but also to the face. Regular gymnastic mimic exercises strengthen the elasticity of the skin and make the face firmer.

❖ With your middle finger, stroke the line from the corner of your mouth to the base of your nose, sharpening your lips.

❖ To smooth the frown line, place your hands on your forehead so that the ball of your thumb touches the brows and push the skin up while facing the ground.

HEADLONG

Many Hollywood stars also swear by this anti-ageing method. The head posture promotes blood circulation in the face and scalp and at the same time strengthens the abdominal and neck muscles for a firmer silhouette.

CLOSING STATEMENT

I hope this book has inspired you and your future culinary life will be enriched with a lot of collagen. You will certainly feel a difference and your health will thank you for it.

Please rate my book on Amazon.de, a short review will do.

Your Melanie Krinz

Imprint

Author: Melanie Krinz

copyright

Author: Melanie Krinz

Title: The Collagen Diet

© by Melanie Krinz, 2018

self publishing

melanie.krinz@yahoo.de

Printed in Great Britain
by Amazon